Bone Broth

Feel Young and Healthier in 30 Days

Table of Contents

Introduction

We all want to feel better, get healthier, and look younger, but that's a lot easier said than done in today's world. Why? Because we are all so harassed with chemicals, toxins, hard work, and lack of sleep. Not exactly the makings for a youthful glow.

Anything you can do to make yourself feel better and look younger is a welcome idea in your life, and bone broth is one of the easiest ways you can do this. Bone broth has been around for centuries, and there's little wonder as to why. When you are able to incorporate this into your life on a regular basis, you are going to see a lot of wonderful results appear in a matter of days.

You will feel better, have healthier skin, and embrace a youthful glow that will stick with you throughout your day. This is going to help you lose those last few pounds that you have been wanting to lose, as well as strengthen your immune system.

You can't beat the benefits that come from the use of bone broth, and once you realize how fast and easy it is to make, you won't ever go back. Bone broth is one of the most nutrient dense things you can have in your fridge, and once you add it to your dishes, you are going to drum up the nutrients and not pack on the calories.

This is the perfect combination for anyone that wants to increase the nutrition in their diet but not the calories. This is going to help you gain all of the benefits and not have to sacrifice on your caloric intake. You don't have to stress about the calories in it, because there are so few, yet you will certainly see the good results.

Bone broth is so easy to make, and there are so many ways you can use it you won't have a problem working it into your day. You can use the guide in this book to make the best bone broth possible, and you can use the bone broth you make in so many ways you won't have to stress about getting it into your diet as you may with some of the other healthy things.

Bone broth has been around for centuries, and it won't take long before you see why. Get ready to discover and ancient art that is going to change the way you cook, eat, and take care of yourself for good!

Chapter 1 – An Overview on Bone Broth

Whenever you want to try something new, you have to get a feel for what it is about. If you don't understand the why behind the method, how are you going to know for sure if it is going to work or not?

With this book, I want to give you that overview first, so you know just what you're dealing with, and how you can use it to get the best results you can imagine.

Are you ready?

You are about to enter the world of bone broth, and I guarantee you will love the results so much, you won't ever go back to another kind of broth again.

What is it?

Bone broth is a substance that has been around for thousands of years. It was very popular in the Far East and Middle Eastern countries, as they were dedicated to using the entire animal in their preparations.

In its most basic form, bone broth is a broth that is made using the bones of an animal. There may be meat with the bones, or there may not, but there is largely just the bones.

Bone broth is the best way you can use the entire animal without getting stuck on how to use the bones. Bone is a hard thing to work with, mainly because it is really hard. You can't cut it up, you can't eat it as is, and it is nearly impossible to get the marrow out of it.

With bone broth, you can soften the bones to the point where you can use them as they are, no matter what the animal is they come from. You can even use fish for a saltier bone broth, even if it is a small batch!

What kind of broths are out there?

Any animal you can get bones from, you can also get bone broth from. Poultry broth is very popular, as is beef, pork, and fish. Poultry and fish are more common in the Orient, while beef is more popular out in the Western countries.

You can even make combination broths if you would like. Be careful what you put together with this, though, as you can mix bones that aren't the best tasting together.

Try to keep beef and pork on their own, but you can use duck and chicken bones together. It is going to take some time and experience before you know just what you want. There's no shame in trial and error.

Once you know what you like, use that. Follow the recipes and see what you want to use as your base bone, and experiment from there with the different veggies you can use to bring out the best flavor.

Why is bone broth so good for health?

Bones are full of all kinds of nutrients that we don't recognize at first, but if you look closer, you will notice that there is a plethora of benefits. Bones are hard to eat as is, but if you boil them in water, you end up with a broth that is full of all of the benefits of the bones, but in liquid form.

With the ease of use and the benefits, bone broth is one of the easiest things to use in a weight loss plan as well as health.

Chapter 2 – Best Bone Broth Benefits

As I mentioned in the last chapter, there are all kinds of benefits of that come with bone broth. This is one of those things that you can use in a variety of ways, and get the other benefits along with it.

If you are eating the bone broth for your weight loss, you are going to have youthful skin and great skin and hair. If you are doing this for the healthy benefits, you are going to slim down and reach a healthy weight.

But, we should take a look at the benefits in particular. What exactly it is that helps you and why, and how you can better use the benefits for your health.

Now, I want to take a look at what those benefits are.

Why using bone broth is your secret to success

There are a number of ways people tell you to lose weight. Or to get rid of the wrinkles in your skin. Or to have more shine in your hair or stronger nails.

Bone broth is a concentrated form of the nutrients you find in the meat. When you use bone broth, you can incorporate the concentrated nutrition into your dishes without adding all the bulk.

Whether you want to use bone broth for your fasting days, or if you want to add a splash to the meals you are making, you are going to have all of your issues solved with bone broth.

Bone broth and weight loss

Why does bone broth help with weight loss? The results are double. Not only does bone broth keep you full with little calories, it will also increase your metabolism, which means it jump starts your weight loss plan.

When you incorporate bone broth into your diet on a regular basis, along with taking bone broth fasts, you are going to lose weight so quickly, you won't even realize you are before you are at your goal.

One of the reasons bone broth also helps with weight loss is because bone broth is filling. It leaves you feeling satisfied without adding a lot of calories and virtually no fat. This means that you can indulge all you want and still lose the weight in a short amount of time.

Not to mention that with this added energy you are going to be able to work out well. Giving all your effort into the workout is going to maximize your calorie burn as well as boost your energy throughout the day. The combination of this is what is going to make you feel younger and more vibrant throughout your day.

Bone broth and your youth

In addition to the energy that bone broth gives you, bone broth is full of awesome benefits… including a high amount of natural gelatin. This gelatin comes from the joints and knuckles, and it helps your stomach and your own joints.

If you add this into your diet on a regular basis, you will forget the problems you have with your stomach, and you can say goodbye to the achy joints. Chondroitin Sulfate… another aspect that you find in bone broth is not only going to help the joints you have as they are, but it is also going to prevent you from getting osteoporosis.

What could be better for your bones than bones, after all? Everything you need to keep your bones healthy and strong is going to be found in the bones that you put into this broth, which means that you will get all of the bone benefits from the broth itself.

We can credit this strength to your bones to the Phosphorous Magnesium that you find in the bones. And, it goes without saying that the calcium is going to do its work in your body.

All in all, if you add bone broth to your diet, you are going to feel the younger frame inside of you that you enjoyed in your youth. You can say goodbye to the shaking joints, the creaking bones, the aches and pains as you sit down and stand up.

While there isn't a definite reason for the energy that comes along with this broth, everyone that has ever tried it swears that you will love the energetic results.

Bone broth for a healthier you

You may be surprised to hear that a lot of the issues you have in your body comes through your gut. Your intestines and stomach do so much for your health that you don't realize when you feel well. We all think that if we have a stomach ache, we must be sick, but if we don't, we're fine.

That's not actually true. You can have different kinds of stomach issues that you don't even realize, because you don't have a stomach ache with them. You may have tiny holes or lesions in the sides of your stomach, or in the walls of your intestines, that could cause you immunity issues, digestive issues, and a wealth of other problems.

Bone broth has a lot of gelatin in it that plugs these holes. It helps you heal, literally from the inside out. If you use it often enough, you not only are going to cure any issue that you currently have, but you will prevent any further issues from developing.

Prevention is always the best cure. This is a truth that has been known for a long time.

Not only does this heal the issues you do have, but it helps prevent other problems in the future

Inflammation, infections, and fragile bones are all issues that most people struggle with as they age. The older you get, the more your bones are going to break down and become bitter.

If you use bone broth often, you are going to slow down the deterioration of your bones, as well as soothe the inflammations you can have. Infections are another common ailment that comes along with age, but bone broth inhibits infections of all kinds.

If you can prevent yourself from ever getting an infection, you can prevent a lot of the other issues that come along with it. The more you are able to do this, the healthier you will be.

Chapter 3 – Your Weight Loss Plan

Obviously, weight loss is one of the main reasons people these days indulge in the bone broth diet. You can, of course, do this for other reasons besides weight loss, and if you do, you will have weight loss as a wonderful side effect, but for those of you that want to use bone broth to lose weight, this chapter is for you.

I have put together this bone broth weight loss plan that is going to give you the results you are after, and fast. One month or less, and you will slim down and feel better. You may not reach your goal in just a month, but you are definitely going to lose a lot of that weight you have been wanting to.

This is going to get you to your goal, and fast. If you don't reach your goal in a month, you are going to in just a few weeks more. There's no way you can be on this diet and not lose the weight, so don't stress about it. Follow the diet plan and exercise, and you are going to reach your goals.

The method behind the madness

If you want to lose weight, you have to remember that the only healthy way to do that is to exercise regularly. You don't have to spend hours in the gym, but you should get your heart rate up for roughly 20 minutes a day a few days a week.

In addition to that, you need to use a healthy diet to help you get to your goals, and bone broth is a great way to do that.

You can add bone broth to your meals as is, or you can base your meals around bone broth. There are even days you can dedicate to bone broth and use that as your primary source for those days.

For maximum results, you need to alternate your broth days with regular days, especially if you want to ensure the best results that will stick.

Think about it, you aren't going to want to live off of broth for the rest of your life. The holidays, date nights, and other events are going to make it nearly impossible to stick to broth all the time. But, you can get even better results if you alternate the days you use the broth with days that you don't.

And even on your off days you can use broth to some extent. I am going to show you the best way to combine the fasting with the non-fasting, and incorporate a real life diet plan that you can stick with for long term. This is a way of life, and if you do it, you are going to get all of the great benefits that you are looking for.

Fasting days

On a typical bone broth diet, you are going to see that there are days when you fast, and there are days when you don't. Some bone broth diets encourage you to eat bone broth primarily, with few deviations from the broth.

I disagree with this mindset. I think you are going to get better, long lasting results if you were to use bone broth intermittently, and add it into the diet you are already eating. You don't have to give up on all the foods you love, but you do have to switch it up a bit if you want to get the best results.

The one thing you need to get used to is the fasting. Fasting days are the days when you use bone broth almost exclusively.

To do this effectively, you need to use bone broth… and only bone broth… as your meal. You are going to make all kinds of broths with a variety of meats and veggies, so you don't have to worry about getting tired of the meal plan.

One of the reasons so many people give up on this is because they don't make the variety that they should with their broths. This means they get so caught up in their one kind of broth, they neglect to make more. This is going to become mundane and boring fast, which makes living off of this broth for an extended period of time dreadful… making it less likely you will stick with it.

Now, let's get back to the fasting in general. Fasting days are singular days you take when you want to lose weight. You are going to focus on just your bone broth during these days, meaning that you don't eat any solids.

You only do single days at a time. I know there are plans that keep you on the bone broth for up to a week at a time, but I don't think that's at all necessary for you to lose the weight. In fact, I think it is better all around for you and your weight loss if you were to take a singular fasting day at a time.

The reason for this is because our bodies are designed to use solids. Your body wants to get nutrients from solids. That's why we have the teeth we have, and the primary diets we have. If you can, however, mix and match your fasting days with your solid days, you're going to get maximum results.

The day of your fast

The day is really quite simple. You replace your meals with bone broth. You can do this by either drinking it, eating it like soup (only the broth), or heating it and drinking it as tea.

Let me assure you, it is a lot easier to get it down if you heat it and eat it like tea or soup, but there are those that like to consume it cold. Drink plenty of water and your broth… as much as you want. I don't think you need to limit yourself on your fasting days, just that you are sticking to your broth exclusively.

Intermittent fasting

So what do I mean by intermittent fasting? All this means is that you take your fasting days regularly. You don't do it every day, but you don't do it randomly, either. You just take your day regularly, and leave it at that.

I suggest that you take a bone broth fasting day twice a week. Try doing it on Saturday and Tuesday or Sunday and Wednesday. If you do it these days, you are going to be doing it as evenly distributed as possible, yet frequently enough that you can still plan your life around it.

The more of a schedule you can get on, the more you can stick with it, and the better results you are going to have.

Stick with it for the long run

There are two main things you need to keep in mind if you are going to have success. The first thing is that a schedule is the key to success. When you know what to plan on, you know what to expect. This means you can plan your life around it, and you can stick with it.

The other thing you need to keep in mind is the fact life happens. You can loosen up and take days off here and there. You can skip days, or you can move them around. The more flexibility you add into your schedule, the more likely you will be to stick with it.

The reason I say this is because you can't fail at this. I hear so many people say they ruined their diet, and they failed at their plan. I am trying to set this up as a way of life for you, which means you can't do it wrong. If you are flexible, and you are willing to pick yourself up if you skip a day, then you will get it for the long run.

Think of it this way: You can't fail at going to work. You may call in sick one day, you may have other reasons that you can't go to work, but that doesn't make you fail at your job.

All you do is go back to work the next day you can. You don't stress about it, you don't worry about it, and you don't stress, you don't give up. You get up, you go back to work, and you go on just like nothing ever happened.

This is because your work is part of your life. You don't consider it failing if you happen to take a day off here and there, and the same goes for your diet. If you are consistent, you are going to reach your goal.

That's how it works. And you can't fail at your diet, just like you can't fail at your life. So, don't worry about it. Take your fast days, take your non-fasting days, and see the awesome benefits come out.

Chapter 4 – How to Make Bone Broth

Now, we get down to the fun part. It's time to make your very own bone broth!

There are a lot of variations you can do with these recipes, so don't be afraid to mix and match the bones you use in the recipes.

Remember if you use fish, you can put in the heads and fins as well as the bones, and make sure you are careful to strain out the solids. There can be a few stray bones if you aren't careful, so always be on the watch for those!

Have fun with it and see what bones you like the best, and you won't ever have an issue with coming up with a broth to use.

Bone broth basic recipe

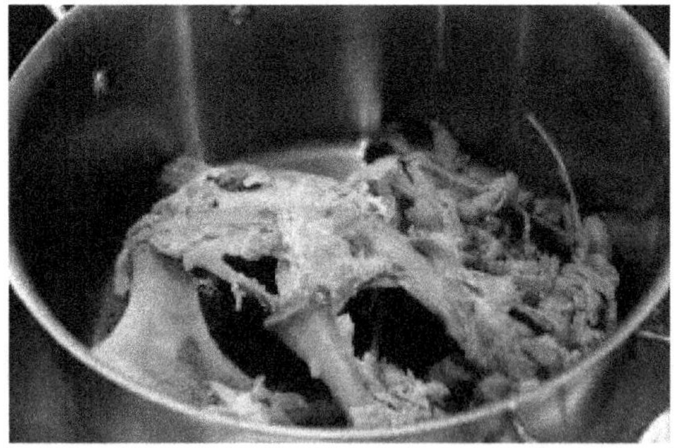

1 large onion

Salt

Pepper

5 carrots

5 celery stalks

2 pounds bird bones of your choice

Boil in a large pot for 18 hours, or until the bones are soft enough to crumble. Leave on the foam that rises to the top, there is a lot of nutrition in this that you can mix in later on.

If you really don't like the foam, you can skim it off, there is still a lot of the nutrition in the broth, but I still recommend that you leave it on.

Easy Peasy Bone Broth

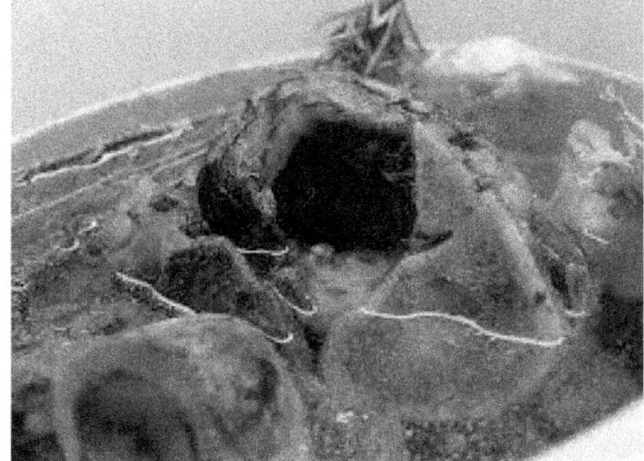

2 pounds beef bones

1 package frozen peas

Garlic

Salt

Pepper

1 onion

2 celery stalks

Boil in a large pot for 18 hours, or until the bones are soft enough to crumble. Leave on the foam that rises to the top, there is a lot of nutrition in this that you can mix in later on.

If you really don't like the foam, you can skim it off, there is still a lot of the nutrition in the broth, but I still recommend that you leave it on.

Bone broth for every palate

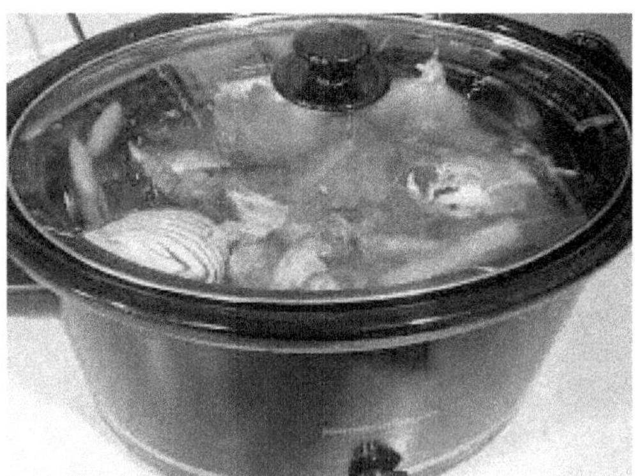

2 pounds fish bones

Salt

Pepper

3 green onions

Garlic

Parsley

Lemon zest

Boil in a large pot for 18 hours, or until the bones are soft enough to crumble. Leave on the foam that rises to the top, there is a lot of nutrition in this that you can mix in later on.

If you really don't like the foam, you can skim it off, there is still a lot of the nutrition in the broth, but I still recommend that you leave it on.

Common mistakes to avoid making your bone broth

The biggest mistake that you can make with bone broth is not letting it boil long enough. You need to let it sit there for hours, or even days if you want to get the best results.

If you're not sure if the bone broth is done, touch the bones. You want them to be so soft they fall apart under your touch. When they are this soft, you are ready to strain them out.

The next most common mistake that people make with their bone broth is to over season or under season it. You want to put in the amount of seasons you like. Maybe that's a lot, maybe it's only a little bit.

When you are happy with it, you know it's ready. Don't get trapped in the thinking that there's only one right way to do it. There is a lot of room for variation, and if you are able to embrace that, you are ready to make it any way you want.

Store your bone broth properly

Bone broth can be stored in glass jars in the fridge for up to 2 weeks, and in the freezer for up to 6 weeks. It is very important that you don't use bone broth that is past its prime, so make sure you use it up quickly.

Your bone broth is going to be the best thing for your diet, as long as you get it in its prime.

Chapter 5 – How to Use Bone Broth for Weight Loss and Youth

I could put in specific recipes for you to follow, but I feel that it is a very limiting way to do it. If you want to use bone broth to lose weight, then you need to put it into your life as it is.

The easiest way to do this is to swap out the bone broth for other things you use in your day to day cooking. Use bone broth in your soups as the base instead of water. Or, you can mix bone broth with a bit of water to dilute it down to your own preference.

If you are cooking rice or pasta, add in a couple tablespoons to the water you are using. This is going to give your pasta and broth a fuller flavor, and make it feel more filling as you eat it. Suddenly, you can eat rice as a meal, instead of needing to put all of these things into it to make it taste better.

You can braise your veggies in it to give them that kick you have always wanted and feel like is missing. You can add it to your gravies and even to the meat you are using. Use it as a marinade for your favorite steaks or roasts for added benefits, and for fuller flavor.

When you see all the benefits start to come into play, you will want to add it to everything you are eating, and I'm telling you now that's ok! You can put it in anything you like, and remember to use it in your fasting days as is. Throw in a fasting day here and there, and you won't feel like all you eat is bone broth, even if you put it into all of your other dishes.

Remember that this is part of your life now, which means that you can still live your life as you want, but with bone broth added in. I know you are going to fall in love with the results as well as the broth itself, so have fun with it and see what comes to your own mind!

Conclusion

There you have it, everything you need to know about bone broth, and all of what you need to make it the best you can. You are going to love all of the ways you can use bone broth, and how easy it is to make.

I want you to remember that this is a process, and you are going to have to work at it if you want to make it the best it can be. There are those that say they have to work at it for a while before they are able to get the results that they want. You are going to have to put in the time and effort for you to get just what you want.

One of the biggest mistakes beginners make when they are making bone broth is the fact they rush the process, and they don't work with the results. You can follow all of the recipes you want, but if you don't like the results, you aren't going to want to make it.

Go ahead and twist and tweak until you get just what you want, and you are going to be hooked on the delicious bone broth you make. What will make it even better is that you can use it in so many ways and for so many different recipes, this is not at all a dish that is going to make you feel stuck.

So what are you waiting for? There are all kinds of bone broths out there just waiting for you to try your hand at them, and once you discover the world that awaits you, you will never want to go back to anything else again.

FREE Bonus Reminder

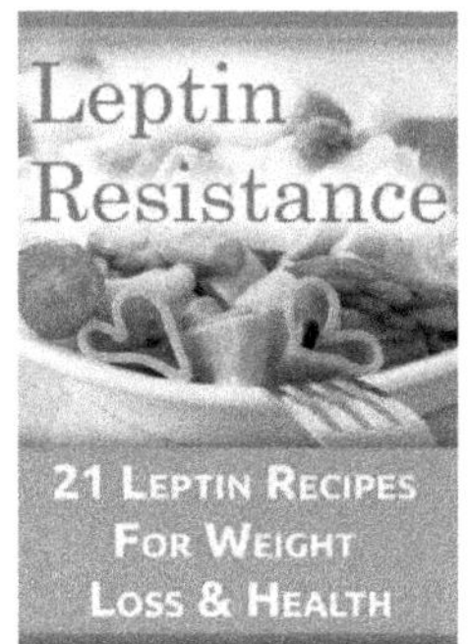

If you have not grabbed it yet, please go ahead and download your special bonus report *"Leptin Resistance. 21 Leptin Recipes For Weight Loss & Healthy Living"*.

Simply Click the Button Below

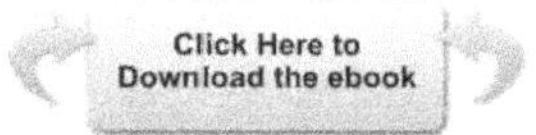

OR **Go to This Page**

http://easyweightlossway.com/free/

BONUS #2: More Free & Discounted Books

Do you want to receive more Free & Discounted Books?

We have a mailing list where we send out our new Books when they go free or with a discount on Kindle. Click on the link below to sign up for Free & Discount Book Promotions.

=> Sign Up for Free & Discount Book Promotions <=

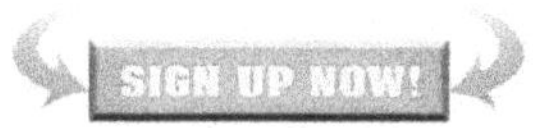

OR Go to this URL

http://zbit.ly/1WBb1Ek

www.ingramcontent.com/pod-product-compliance
Lightning Source LLC
Chambersburg PA
CBHW061929270726
48660CB00003BA/1114